Francisca Elineuda Morais Martins
Camila A. Sousa Silva
Nayara C. R. Oliveira

Motorcyclists Victims of Traffic Accidents

Francisca Elineuda Morais Martins
Camila A. Sousa Silva
Nayara C. R. Oliveira

Motorcyclists Victims of Traffic Accidents

Epidemiological profile of patients treated at a referral hospital in the city of Parnaíba-PI

ScienciaScripts

This book is a translation from the original published under ISBN 978-613-9-62426-3.

Publisher:
Sciencia Scripts
is a trademark of
Dodo Books Indian Ocean Ltd. and OmniScriptum S.R.L publishing group

120 High Road, East Finchley, London, N2 9ED, United Kingdom
Str. Armeneasca 28/1, office 1, Chisinau MD-2012, Republic of Moldova, Europe
Printed at: see last page
ISBN: 978-620-7-72502-1

SUMMARY

"That's exactly what life is made of, moments.

Moments that we have to go through, whether good or bad, for our own learning. Never forgetting the most important thing: Nothing in this life is by chance.

Absolutely nothing. So we have to worry about doing our bit, as best we can.

Life doesn't always follow our will, but it is perfect in what it has to be." Chico Xavier

SUMMARY

In Brazil and around the world, lives are interrupted due to the large number of traffic accidents that occur every day. In view of the above, it is necessary to trace the epidemiological profile of motorcyclists treated at the Reference Hospital in the municipality of Parnaiba-PI, in addition to characterizing the socio-demographic profile of the victims; determining the most injured body area, the type of injury produced and the possible sequelae of the accidents. This is a descriptive, exploratory study with a quantitative approach. The setting for the study was a public referral hospital, with a sample of 109 victims of motorcycle accidents. Data was collected from January to February 2015, after which it was tabulated in a Microsoft Excel spreadsheet in order to organize and construct graphs and tables. It was found that most of the victims were men, young people aged between 21 and 30, single, with incomplete primary education and a family income of between one and two minimum wages. Most of the motorcyclists involved in accidents were drivers and did not have a National Driver's License, and the main cause of the accidents was the use of alcoholic beverages. Identifying this data shows the local reality, which can have serious consequences. Among the measures found and cited to reduce this alarming number of victims of motorcycle accidents is a joint effort between the education, health, justice and traffic sectors.

Keywords: Accidents. Trauma. Injury. Helmets.

1   INITIAL CONSIDERATIONS

In Brazil and around the world, lives are disrupted due to the large number of traffic accidents that occur every day. In many cases, even if there is no fatality, families have their routine affected and transformed by the impact of an accident. It's not just the physical after-effects, but also the psychological, social and economic ones.

Studies released in 2010 and 2013 by the World Health Organization, for the formulation and support of the 2013 Map of Violence, indicate staggering figures of a serious lethal epidemic in road traffic on the planet. In 2010 alone, there were 1.24 million deaths from traffic accidents in 182 countries around the world. Between 20 and 50 million survive with trauma and injuries. Today, these accidents already represent a global cost of US$ 518 billion/year. If nothing is done, the WHO estimates that there will be 1.9 million traffic deaths in 2020 and 2.4 million in 2030 (WAISELFISZ, 2013).

The epidemiological profile of traffic in Piaui, according to DETRAN-PI, recorded 10,517 traffic accidents with and without victims in the state in 2010. The state's vehicle fleet totaled 583,050. The State Highway Police Battalion (BPRE) also recorded 1554 traffic offenses, the most common of which were: driving a vehicle with altered lighting/signaling equipment; driving in the opposite direction on a one-way street; driving a vehicle with a size/load greater than the established limit. The city of Parnaiba had a fleet of 46,971 vehicles and the number of accidents with victims was 291, of which 24 were fatal (DETRAN-PI, 2010).

For the Ministry of Health, a transport accident is any accident involving a vehicle intended, or used at the time of the accident, primarily for transporting people or goods from one place to another. A traffic accident is any accident involving a vehicle on a public road, originating, ending or involving a vehicle partially situated on the public road. A motorcyclist is considered to be any person traveling on a motorcycle or in a sidecar or trailer attached to this vehicle (BRASIL, 2008).

Motorcycles are increasingly being used for both work and leisure. The tendency for cities to swell exponentially could lead to an increase in the number of accidents of this type, due to the constant competition in chaotic traffic (GOLIAS, 2013).

This statistic has an economic impact (costs), as the government spends a huge amount on surgery, rehabilitation and pensions, among other things. In 2010, SUS spent a total of R$187 million on hospitalizations due to traffic accidents. Spending on hospitalizations for motorcyclists was R$ 43.9 million in 2007 (37% of the total). These costs almost doubled in 2010: R$ 85.5 million (45% of the total costs). (ASDECOM-DETRAN-PA).

In view of the high global and regional rates of morbidity and mortality caused by traffic accidents, policies have been implemented to prevent these diseases. In 2001, the National Policy for the Reduction of Morbidity and Mortality from Accidents and Violence was approved, the fundamental purpose of which is to reduce morbidity and mortality from accidents and violence in the country. These interventions are aimed at developing a set of articulated and systematized actions in order to contribute to the population's quality of life (BRASIL, 2001).

In 2002, the Project for the Reduction of Morbidity and Mortality from Traffic Accidents was also launched with the aim of implementing health promotion actions through the articulation and mobilization of governmental and non-governmental sectors and the population in general (SECRETARIA DE POLITICAS DE SAUDE/MS, 2002).

This panorama allows us to visualize a better quality of life for motorcyclists, and it is necessary to adopt and implement existing public policies to combat the morbidity and mortality of these victims. This work must be articulated between the sectors of Education, Health, Justice, among others.

Faced with this reality, we chose as the object of this study motorcyclists who were victims of traffic accidents, treated at a hospital in the city of Parnaiba-Piaui. The topic was chosen as a result of our experiences during the undergraduate course. I saw the need to deepen my knowledge of the population who are victims of traffic accidents, especially motorcyclists, because this is the most used means of transportation in the city of Parnaiba and the region, as well as being a major cause of death and disability in the world.

In view of the above and considering the WHO guidelines, in order for there to be training, rehabilitation and education that promote safe and preventive behavior in traffic, based on the serious and innumerable consequences of traffic accidents (TA) and the high social cost, it is necessary to know the socio-cultural context in which a given population lives. Therefore, this data will serve as a basis for the local reality, highlighting the need to adopt urgent measures to effectively combat traffic accidents.

2 OBJECTIVES

2.1 General Objective

- To trace the epidemiological profile of motorcyclists, victims of traffic accidents, treated at the reference hospital in the municipality of Parnaiba-PI.

2.2 Specific Objectives

- To characterize the sociodemographic profile of car accident victims;

- Identify the main factors that cause accidents involving motorcyclists;

- To describe the most prevalent characteristics of motorcyclists who have been victims of accidents, such as: type of victim, driver's license, length of driver's license, drug use, use of protective equipment, previous accidents;

- To determine the most injured body area, the type of injury produced and the possible sequelae of motorcycle accidents.

3 THEORETICAL FRAMEWORK

3.1 Historical Context

The high number of vehicles, related to the purchasing power of the population, increases the ease of purchase in production, this fact cannot be considered as the only cause of accidents, since it can be associated with the existence of a relationship with the increase in the number of accidents, the acquisition of the motorcycle becoming a reality in the social context (TDR- MOBILITY PLAN, 2012).

The use of this vehicle (motorcycle) has been expanding due to the fact that it is a very agile and cheaper vehicle than the car, and its use is not only for leisure, but mainly as a means of transportation to work (ANDRADE, 2001).

In 2012, Brazil had a total fleet of 76,137,125 motor vehicles. The number of cars rose from just over 24.5 million in 2001 to 50.2 million in 2012. Over the years there has been a reduction in the number of cars and a considerable increase in the motorcycle fleet. In 2001, motorcycles accounted for 14.2% of all motor vehicles and by the end of 2012, they accounted for 26.2%. The Northeast experienced a considerable increase in the motorization rate between 2001 and 2012, from 5.3 to 11.1 (RODRIGUES, 2013).

According to data from DENATRAN, in 2014 the accumulated vehicle fleet in the state of Piaui in 2002 was 24,927. In 2013 this figure rose to 90,659 of the total number of vehicles in the entire state. In June 2014, only 24,232 were registered, a figure that compared to 2002 represented the whole. In that month and year, the city of Parnaiba had a vehicle fleet of 68,195. Of this total, motorcycles accounted for 34,558, representing more than 50% of all vehicles registered during the month of June.

The exorbitant growth in the number of motorcycles compared to cars; not only as an instrument of easy access and also justified by their effectiveness in driving, motorcycles have over the years become a real source of problems and chaos for health services. It is the little or no perception of risk that has led to the strong adherence to motorcycles, which is worth emphasizing how much prevention work is needed for motorcyclists, and should be included from the purchase of the vehicle to daily use on public roads (ROCHA, 2013).

3.2 Epidemiology

A recent study carried out by the World Health Organization (WHO) with 181 countries, which summarizes the number of deaths and rates (per 100,000 inhabitants) of traffic fatalities, places Brazil in 33rd place. A second study of 122 countries, which presents the mortality rate for two- and three-wheeled motor vehicles, places Brazil in 13th position among the 122 countries listed (WAISELFISZ, 2013).

In 2011, 66.6% - two thirds - of traffic victims were pedestrians, cyclists and/or motorcyclists, but the national trends of the last decade are showing a marked difference to the rest of the world, with a heavy increase in the lethality of motorcyclists. Motorcycles have become the focal point and explanatory cause of the growth in our daily mortality on public roads. In 10 of the 27 OECD (Organization for Economic Cooperation and Development) countries, the number of motorcyclists killed has increased, and in Brazil this increase has been 275% in this category (WAISELFISZ, 2013).

A survey carried out in the city of Parnaiba showed that from January to June 2010, the main types of accident were collisions (42.9%), motorcycle crashes (30.2%) and being run over (14.4%). In terms of the vehicles involved, motorcycles (65.7%) and cars (16.1%) stand out (PRADO, 2011).

A second study shows the main victims of traffic accidents and shows that motorcycle occupants are significantly the most affected in these occurrences, with 839 cases, corresponding to 70.92%. Car occupants, on the other hand, are the second most affected group of victims, with 164 occurrences recorded in the period surveyed, corresponding to 13.86% of cases (SILVA, 2013).

3.3 Characterization of traffic accidents

Movement injuries are responsible for the majority of deaths and injuries in our country. The higher the speed, the greater the energy, and consequently the more serious the injuries. In a sudden deceleration or collision at 100 km/h, the body weighs 28 times more. We call it closed trauma when there is a deformity of the external part that returns to normal leaving internal damage. Organs such as the spleen and liver can be ruptured without the injury being externalized. In penetrating trauma, a permanent cavity is formed. On motorcycles we have a collision followed by a fall (ALVES JR, 2014).

According to NBR 10.697, of June 1980, from the Brazilian Association of Technical Standards (ABNT), accidents are conceptualized and classified as follows: Collision: an accident in which there is an impact between moving vehicles; Crash: the impact of a moving vehicle against any fixed obstacle; Lock-up: a rear-end collision involving three or more vehicles; Run-over: an accident in which a pedestrian or animal is hit by a motorized or non-motorized vehicle; Other: an accident in which a pedestrian or animal is hit by a motorized or non-motorized vehicle (BRASIL-MT, 2002).

We must consider that speed is more important than mass. Doubling the mass of the car will double the energy, while doubling the speed will quadruple the energy. A collision at 60 km/h represents a fall from the 11th floor of a building. At 80 km/h it would be from the 20th floor (ALVES JR, 2014).

In a study carried out in the south of Brazil, motorcyclists suffered injuries ranging from traumatic brain injuries to spinal cord injuries, which were considered extremely serious, including limb amputations; lower and upper limb fractures; and various injuries and dislocations. Of all the amputations, 94.6% were of the lower limb, affecting the tibia and/or hip joint. The rest were lower limb extremities (foot or calcaneus) or hand and arm (SCHOELLER, 2012).

According to Santos (2008), the occurrence of sequelae was identified in all the body areas surveyed in a given study. It should be noted that of the 49.5% of accident victims with sequelae, 80.7% had temporary sequelae and 19.2% had permanent sequelae.

3.4 Measures to reduce the number of traffic accidents

In several countries, the loss of human life in traffic is becoming increasingly controlled. Some nations, such as Sweden, have managed to set a target of zero traffic deaths. All scholars on the subject are unanimous in showing that this kind of goal depends on several factors (NJAINE, 2009).

According to the author, several points can be controlled to reduce the number of traffic victims, such as: Problems of engineering and maintenance of roads and streets with potholes, defects in the lanes; problems of vehicle design and safety, where there should be shared responsibility between companies, workshops and drivers to make traffic and transport safer; problems of drivers whose associated factors are alcohol consumption, drowsiness, lack of respect for signs, traffic fights and speeding; and problems of pedestrians who are not the main culprits in accidents, but are the biggest victims.

Studies have shown that the lethality of motorcycle occupants and drivers of heavy transport (buses and trucks) are priority groups for educational and enforcement interventions, and for taking measures to make traffic safer on urban avenues and highways, where most accidents with victims occur (ANDRADE, 2001).

An important point is the implementation of short- and long-term measures, taking into account aspects related to the user, safety equipment and even the vehicle, inspections and punishments for violations. In the long term, there is a need to improve the education of new drivers and a strict enforcement policy, bearing in mind aspects related to speed control and the use of alcohol while driving (ROCHA, 2013).

Traffic education depends on changing the attitudes of both drivers and pedestrians. Traffic rules need to be disseminated in schools, since all pupils are pedestrians and will be driving cars in the future. Part of an individual's development comes from becoming aware of problems and thus changing their behavior. According to Article 74 of the CTB: "Traffic education is everyone's right and a priority duty for the components of the National Traffic System" (BRUNS, 2006) (BRASIL, 2008).

One of the Ministry of Health's proposals is to set targets for reducing the number of accidents in the states. This will be done by investing in improving the quality of emergency care provided by the Mobile Emergency Care Service (SAMU), when professionals are trained to provide quality prehospital care in order to prevent an increase in deaths from accidents (TDR- MOBILITY PLAN, 2012).

Among the policies adopted, the consolidation of the National Policy for the Reduction of Morbidity and Mortality from Accidents and Violence instituted by Ordinance No. 737/GM on May 16, 2001, is essential to the link between various government segments, for the adoption of improvements covering public roads, compliance with laws provided for in the Brazilian Traffic Code - CTB and education as a fundamental part in the prevention of this aggravation (SANTOS, 2013).

The great value of guidance and education with regard to the practices to be observed when driving safely on public roads among the young age group is reinforced, along with all the monitoring and need for action on other factors related to events involving motorcycles (GOLIAS, 2013).

Traffic safety campaigns are aimed at drivers who behave inappropriately, such as talking on their cell phones, not paying attention, drinking alcoholic beverages, among others. They aim to raise awareness among transport users about road conditions, vehicle maintenance, traffic rules, safety tips, recommended speed and levels of aggression (TDR- MOBILITY PLAN, 2012).

4 RESEARCH METHODOLOGY

This is a descriptive, exploratory study with a quantitative approach which enables the systematic collection of numerical information through control conditions and an analysis of the information using statistics (POLIT; BECK; HUNGLER, 2004).

Descriptive research also has as its main objective the establishment of relationships between variables obtained through the use of standardized data collection techniques (FIGUEIREDO, 2008).

According to Gil (2008), descriptive research describes the characteristics of certain populations or phenomena, using standardized data collection techniques such as questionnaires and systematic observation. Exploratory research is characterized by providing greater familiarity with the problem, involving a bibliographical survey, and also takes the form of a case study.

The setting for the research was a public referral hospital in the municipality of Parnaiba-PI. The institution provides care through the Unified Health System (SUS). It has 145 inpatient and observation beds, 16 of which are for the Surgical Clinic and 22 for the Emergency Room, as well as support rooms. The hospital also has other inpatient units: Medical Clinic, Infectious Diseases, Pediatrics, Obstetrics, General Surgery, Intensive Care Unit - ICU, Neonatal Intensive Care Unit - NICU, among others.

As the only hospital in the region offering high and medium complexity services, it is a reference point for the twelve towns that make up the Piaui Coast micro-region and also for the towns in Ceará and Maranhão that border the state of Piaui.

The study population was made up of victims of motorcycle accidents treated in the Emergency Room and admitted to the Surgical Clinic at the Reference Hospital in the city of Parnaiba-PI. The sample consisted of 109 motorcycle accident victims over the age of 18 who agreed to take part in the study and who met the inclusion and exclusion criteria previously determined by the study.

The inclusion criteria were that participants should be over 18 years old, victims of a motorcycle accident and have favorable clinical conditions to answer the data collection instrument. Men and women under the age of 18 and over the age of 60 and/or those with disorientation that prevented them from understanding the questions or answers were excluded.

Data was collected from January to February 2015, using a questionnaire with closed questions, containing socio-demographic variables and clinical data (Appendix A) with questions formulated by the researcher and using the medical records as support for the collection, in order to gather data pertinent to the object of the research. The research took place on alternate days during the week, in one shift, and on Sundays during those months. After explaining the objectives of the work to those in charge of the sector, the medical records were analyzed in the search for inpatients who had been victims of traffic accidents and who met the inclusion criteria. After the medical records had been analyzed, the patient was approached to explain what the research was about and to clarify any possible doubts, and only after the victim had given his consent would the questionnaire be administered.

The sociodemographic variables assessed were gender, age, marital status, schooling and occupational activity. Other variables surveyed were the circumstances of the accident, whether or not safety equipment was used and the relationship between the occurrence of the event and the suspected use of alcohol. The area of the body that was damaged, injuries and sequelae were also investigated, which allowed for a more precise investigation.

After the data was collected, it was tabulated in a Microsoft Excel® spreadsheet in order to organize it and construct graphs and tables, followed by a discussion based on the theoretical framework on the subject. Descriptive statistics were used to analyze the sociodemographic and clinical variables collected, using absolute and simple frequencies with percentage calculations.

The project was approved by the Research Ethics Committee of the Instituto Camillo Filho/ Sociedade Piauiense de Ensino, meeting the standards established by Resolution No. 466/12, which deals with the Norms of Research Involving Human Beings (BRASIL, 2012). CAAE number: 38982914.2.0000.5212.

Participants who agreed to take part voluntarily in the study signed the Free and Informed Consent Form (Appendix C) in two copies: one from the participant and the other from the researcher. In this form, the participants were informed about the nature of the research, its objectives, methods, the guarantee of anonymity and the right to revoke their previous decision to take part at any time.

The researchers undertook to keep the identity of the research participants confidential, in order to avoid future problems with their explanations.

5 RESULTS

This study considered a total of 109 victims of motorcycle accidents who were admitted to the Surgical Clinic and Emergency Room of a Regional Hospital in Parnaiba in January and February 2015.

Table 1- Profile of the study population, following the socio-demographic variables.

Parnaiba (PI), 2015 (n= 109)

Features	n (109)	%
SEX		
Male	83	76,1
Female	26	23,8
AGE RANGE		
18 -20	18	18,5
21 - 30	42	38,5
31 - 40	15	13,7
41 - 50	18	18,5
51 or more	16	14,6
CIVIL STATUS		
Single	53	48,6
Married	27	24,7
Stable union	25	22,9
Viùvo (a)	2	1,8
Divorced	2	1,8
SCHOOLING		
Elementary school incomplete	47	43,1
Complete elementary school	14	12,8
Secondary school incomplete	13	11,9
Completed high school	24	22
Higher Education Incomplete	2	1,8
Higher education completed	1	0,9
Illiterate	8	7,3
FAMILY INCOME		
Up to 1 minimum wage	42	38,5
From 1 to 2 minimum wages	61	55,9
From 3 to 4 minimum wages	5	4,5
From 5 to 6 minimum wages	1	0,9
TOTAL	**109**	**100**

According to the analysis, more than half of the sample studied was male, with 83 men and 26 women. The predominant age group was 21 to 30 years old (38.5%), followed by 18 to 20 year olds and 41 to 50 year olds with the same percentage (18.5%) and motorcyclists aged 51 or over (14.6%) and 31 to 40 year olds (13.7%).

The variable relating to marital status highlights the number of single people, representing 48.6%, followed by the number of married people with 24.7% and people forming a family in a stable union with 22.9%, only 1.8% were widowed or divorced.

Analyzing the data on level of education, we found that the most reported was incomplete primary education (with 43.1%), followed by complete secondary education (with 22%), complete primary education (with 12.8%), followed by incomplete secondary education (11.9%), and to a lesser extent, but still present in the study, illiterate motorcyclists (with 7.3%), incomplete higher education (1.8%) and complete higher education (0.9%).

Considering the family income of the victims, the largest number of people living on 1 to 2 minimum wages was 61, followed by an income of up to 1 minimum wage (42) and a smaller number of people living on 3 to 4 minimum wages (5) and only 1 person living on 5 to 6 minimum wages.

Graph 1: Distribution of motorcycle accidents, by Federative Unit and Municipality. Parnaiba-Pi, 2015.

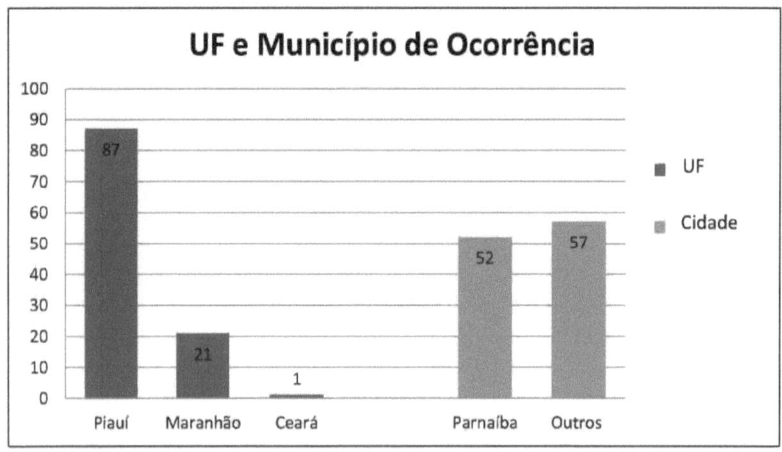

As shown in graph 1, the majority of accidents occurred in the state of Piaui, with 87 cases. Victims from other states were also identified, such as Maranhão (21) and Ceará (1). Of the accidents recorded in the state of Piaui, 52 took place in the city of Parnaiba, while the other 57 were in neighboring towns such as Cocal dos Alves, Luis Correia, Buriti dos Lopes, Caxingó, Bom Principio and others, as shown in the graph.

Graph 2: Distribution of motorcycle accidents, according to the nature of the accidents. Parnaiba-Pi, 2015.

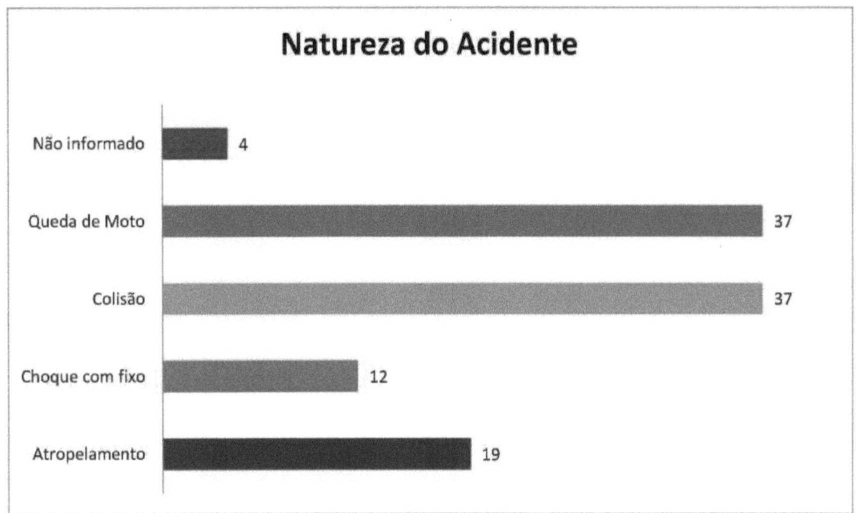

According to the graph above, in the category describing the types of accidents most commonly reported were motorcycle collisions and falls, with 34% of victims, followed by being run over (17.4%) and colliding with a fixed object (11%); and to a lesser extent, 4% of those interviewed did not state the precise nature of the accident.

For the majority of the victims, the main cause of the accidents was alcohol (27%). Some interviewees assumed that they had consumed alcohol before the accident and the others claimed to be victims of third parties who had used alcohol. Also recorded as reasons for the accident were recklessness (22%) and the fault of third parties (18%); problems on the road (14%); mechanical failure (7%) and malpractice (2%). Other causes accounted for 10% of responses, as shown in the graph above.

Graph 3: Distribution of motorcycle accidents, according to the cause of the accident. Parnaiba-Pi, 2015.

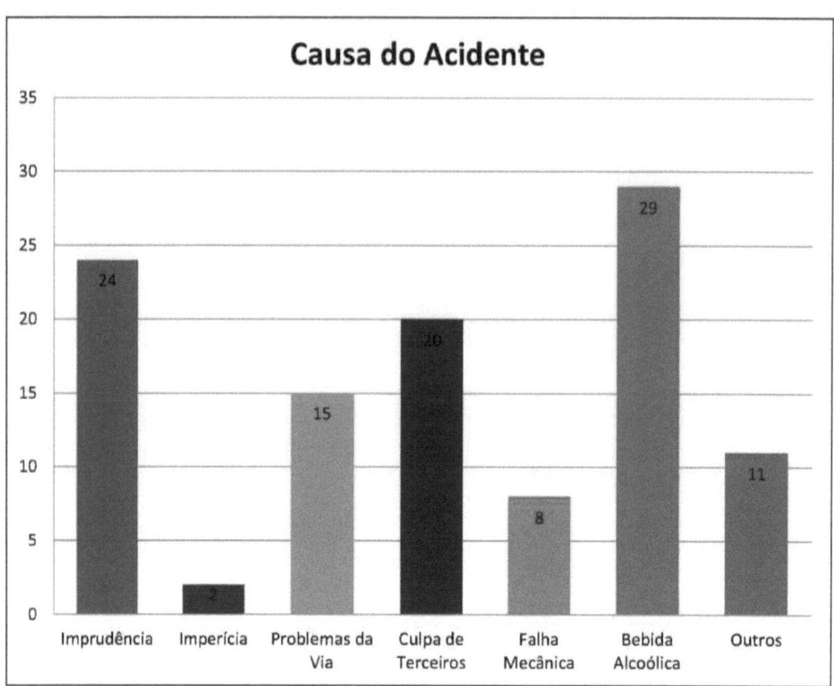

In an attempt to identify the category of victim, a significant proportion of motorcyclists were motorcycle drivers, 67.8% of whom were accident victims, while the remaining 32.1% were passengers.

Of the 74 drivers, only 20% were licensed and the majority (45%) had less than 5 years' driving experience. The range of motorcyclists with the least experience was between 5 and 15 years (35%), followed by more than 20 years licensed (15%) and with the least occurrence in the 16-20 year range (5%), as shown in table 2.

A significant proportion did not drink alcohol, 69.7%. However, the number of people who claimed to have ingested the product is still high, at 28.4%, which is characterized as a crime.

To a lesser extent, but still present in the study, illicit drugs were mentioned by 2 of the interviewees. With regard to helmet use, 55% of motorcyclists reported using PPE (Personal Protective Equipment) and 44.9% did not use it at the time of the accident.

Table 2: Characteristics of individuals treated at the Referral Hospital, according to clinical variables, Parnaiba-Pi, 2015.

Features	n (109)	%
type of victim		

Passenger	35		32,1
Driver	74		67,8
QUALIFIED			
Yes	20		27
No	54		72,9
DRIVING TIME			
Up to 5 years	9		45
5 - 15 years	7		35
16 - 20 years	1		5
More than 20 years	3		15
ALCOHOL/DRUG USE			
Not used	76		69,7
Alcohol	31		28,4
Drugs	2		1,8
WEARING A HELMET			
Yes	60		55
No	49		44,9
PREVIOUS ACCIDENTS			
Yes	50	45,8	
No	59	54,1	
PREVIOUS CA VEHICLE			
Motorcycle	40	80	
Others	10	20	
TOTAL	-	**100**	

The number of individuals who had suffered previous accidents (50) was very close to those who had never had a similar experience (59). However, given the number of victims who have experienced this trauma, the number of repeat motorcycle accidents is notorious and significant, with 80% and only 20% for other types of accidents.

Graph 4 - Distribution of motorcycle accidents according to the injured body region, Parnaiba-Pi, 2015.

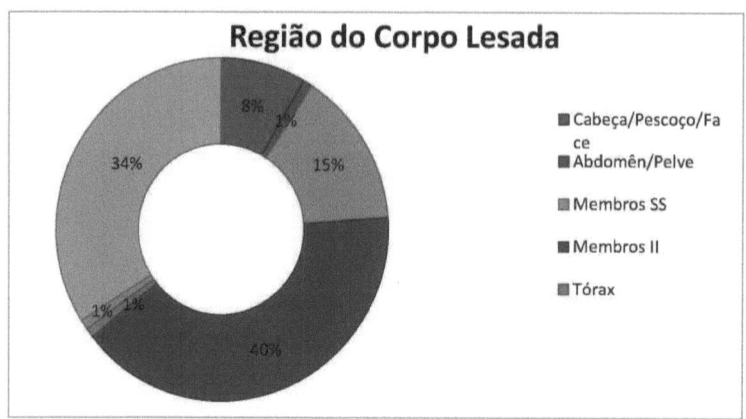

The graph above shows the most affected part of the body: the lower limbs,

including femur, tibia and fibula, with 44 (40.3%) victims. This was followed by polytraumatized victims representing 37 (34%), who suffered not only abrasions but also fractures in various parts of the body. There was less evidence of injuries to the upper limbs with 16 (14.6%) cases; head/neck/face (9%); abdomen/pelvis, thorax and spine with 1 (1%) each.

Graph 5 - Distribution of motorcycle accidents according to type of injury, Parnaiba-Pi, 2015.

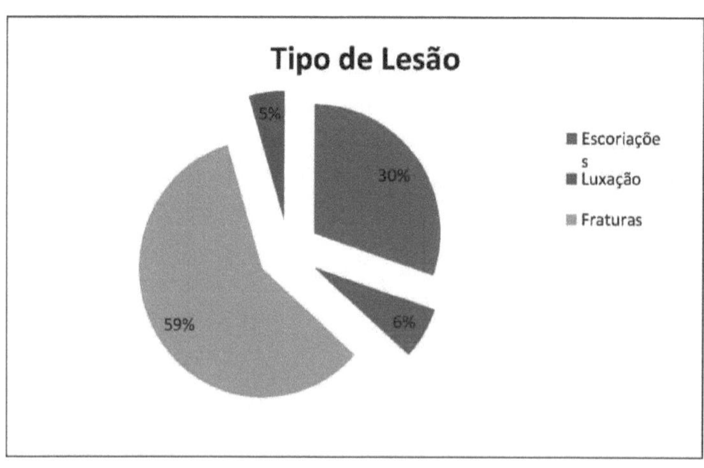

Graph 5 shows the most common traumas recorded in the study: 59% were fractures, followed by 30% of victims with abrasions, 6% had dislocations and 5% were diagnosed with Traumatic Brain Injury (TBI).

Graph 6 - Distribution of motorcycle accidents according to prognosis, Parnaiba-Pi, 2015.

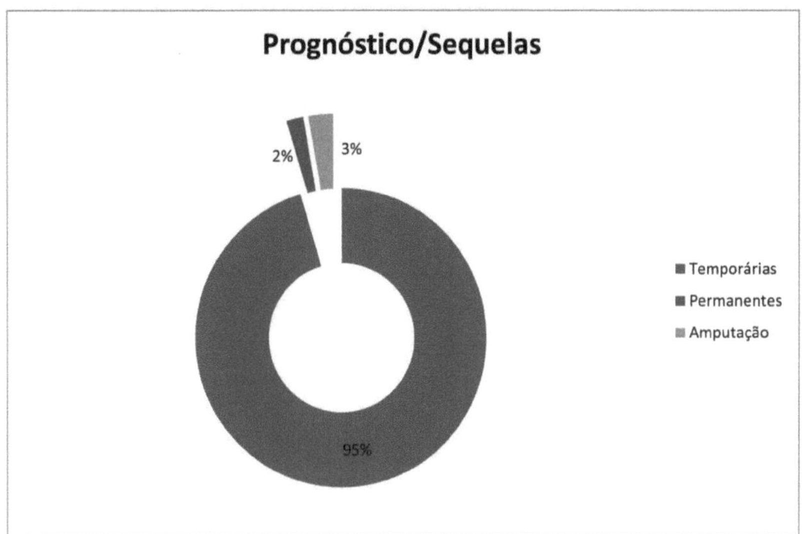

The sequelae of these traumas, according to graph 6, were temporary sequelae with 95% of the records, some of which could take months to recover from, requiring physiotherapy and time off work; 3% of the cases were lower limb amputations and 2% of the victims had permanent sequelae.

6   Discussions

This study, with 109 victims, confirms the reality of small, medium and large cities, where a significant number of traffic accident victims are motorcyclists. In the municipality of São Paulo, 21,795 traffic accidents were reported between 2011 and 2013. Motorcycle accidents accounted for 52.1% and bicycle accidents for 7.1%. With 11,366 motorcycle accidents reported, 16.2% of the victims were pedestrians and 79.1% were the drivers themselves (RODRIGUES, ARMOND, GORIOS et al, 2014).

A second study carried out in the capital Teresina considered a sample of 81 individuals who were admitted to the Teresina Emergency Reference Hospital - PI, victims of motorcycle accidents and who underwent a surgical procedure in May 2014 (NASCIMENTO, 2014).

In the city of Parnaiba, Silva (2014) analyzed 6,741 medical records, of which 1,183 were traffic accidents, corresponding to 17.55% of the SAMU's attendances between January and December 2013. The study showed the main victims of traffic accidents and showed that motorcycle occupants are significantly present in these occurrences, with 839 cases, corresponding to 70.92%. Car occupants are the second most affected group of victims, with 164 occurrences recorded during the study period, corresponding to 13.86% of cases.

According to information from the Parnaiba Health Surveillance, the local Mortality Information System (SIM) recorded 5 deaths from traffic accidents in January and February, 4 of which were motorcycle accidents.

All this data clearly points to the huge proportion that motorcycle accidents have taken on in everyday life. What makes this problem worthy of special attention is precisely the fact that it affects a young, economically active population, who unfortunately still act recklessly, risking their quality of life and well-being due to banal and inconsequential attitudes.

In this study, in relation to the gender of the victim, there was a marked predominance of males, corresponding to 76.1%, compared to 23.8% of females. This large difference may be due to the fact that women are more cautious and pay extra attention when driving a vehicle, as well as being more attentive to details, which is of the utmost importance and can make a difference during a risky situation that requires quicker action.

According to Souza; Mortean; Mendonca (2010), of the 2,683 victims, 71.1% were drivers and 78.1% were male. In the municipality of Campo Mourâo, where the study was carried out, men accounted for 72.38% of the victims in 2005, 65.93% in 2006 and 70.48% in 2007. This corroborates the data from the research carried out by Welter; Frigo; Busnello; et al. (2013), where the highest incidence of victims is male, with 81 male victims and 36 female victims.

Cardoso (2012) concludes in his study that motorcycle falls have a higher incidence in men, due to a factor of greater exposure in traffic, as well as men's more aggressive behavior when it comes to traffic.

Taking into account the age group, a large sample of young people under the age of 18 was observed during data collection, but they were not part of the inclusion criteria, but it should be emphasized that these young people take control of a motorcycle or car with the consent of their parents. Although this is a common practice, it deserves due attention because young people are taking over the driving of dangerous transport such as motorcycles. In this study, young people aged between 21 and 30 predominated, with 38.5%. This confirms the local, regional and Brazilian reality, where a large proportion of young, economically active people are affected. This calls for urgent measures to combat traffic accidents.

Several national studies have found similar results regarding the age group of motorcyclists. Between 2011 and 2013, 21,795 transport accidents were reported in the municipality of São Paulo, with motorcycle accidents accounting for 52.1% and the predominant age group of victims being between 20 and 29 years old, 46.2% (RODRIGUES, 2014).

Oliveira (2012) confirmed in his study that 71.76% of motorcyclists were aged between 20 and 39, with an average age of 27.94. In a study carried out by Mascarenhas (2010), the target population was made up of 30 motorcyclists involved in traffic accidents in the municipality of Jequie/BA, with an average age of 30.93 years, ranging from 17 to 48 years. The results showed that 13 (43.33%) individuals were between 28 and 38 years old.

Duarte (2013) observes that the SAMU advanced support units in Campo Grande - MS, attended to a young population affected by motorcycle accidents, aged between 20 and 29 (44% of cases).

According to Palu (2013), data from 186 patients who were victims of motorcycle accidents were analyzed, of which 93 were married, 85 were single, 7 were separated and only one was widowed. Ferreira (2009) reported that 56% of the motorcyclists analyzed were married and of these, 67% had children.

In the study conducted by Mascarenhas (2010), 19 individuals (63.33%) were single and 10 (33.3%) were married. This situation was also confirmed in this study, where 48.6% of the interviewees were single. We can attribute the greater presence of single victims to the fact that they don't feel the same concern or responsibility as family providers. According to some authors, there is a greater risk of serious or fatal accidents for single people, which can be justified by the fact that single people are more exposed to risk factors (ALMEIDA, 2013).

With regard to the level of education of the victims, Matos (2008) shows a relatively dispersed result: the majority of motorcyclists had completed secondary school (46.2%), followed by those with completed elementary school (28.2%) and only one interviewee with completed higher education (0.9%).

These data were also found in the research carried out by Palu (2013): the majority of victims had a secondary education, 114 (61.3%); followed by primary education, 60 (32.3%) and, to a lesser extent, higher education, with 12 (6.5%) individuals.

A different sample was found by Mascarenhas (2010). He found that 13 (43.33%) of the victims had only incomplete primary education, 7 (23.3%) had incomplete secondary education and 5 (16.6%) had completed secondary education. This result is closer to the reality in the city of Parnaiba, as the majority of the population interviewed had only incomplete primary education, with 43% of the victims, followed by complete secondary education with 22%.

Low levels of education are a determining factor in learning and understanding many situations. We have a population without much education, with a job that offers a basic income and the conditions are not favorable for them to acquire a vehicle that offers greater safety.

With regard to the socio-economic profile of public university students who have been victims of traffic accidents, 60% came from families with an income of more than five minimum wages (MW), 24% from families with an income of three to five MW, 12% from one to three MW, and only one student (0.8%) belonged to a family with an income of less than one MW (IWAMOTO, 2009).

Labiak (2008) also studied young university students, and the average minimum wage was 65.56% (297) of the total number of students with a monthly income of ten minimum wages (MW) or less, and only 7.51% (34) of the students declared an income of more than 21 MW.

A very distant reality from those interviewed, when it comes to the family income of motorcycle accident victims in the city of Parnaiba, who have only 1 to 2 minimum salaries as their income, representing 56%. The vast majority of these riders have a motorcycle as an alternative to public transport, but because it is less expensive and cheaper to maintain, they opt for this less safe alternative.

As for family income, as described by Barros (2008), 279 (75%) motorcyclists had a monthly income of up to 2 minimum wages; 86 (23%) had between three and five minimum wages; and only 5 (1%) had between 6 and 10 minimum wages. Liberatti (2000) states that the poor distribution of income is one of the causes for the population to use low-cost vehicles, stimulating the purchase of motorcycles.

This study shows that the state of Piaui is the federative unit with the highest number of accidents.

The city of Parnaiba accounts for just over 50% of cases. However, it is important to note that Parnaiba is a point of reference for more than ten neighboring cities in terms of advanced medical care. Perhaps this is the reason for the considerable number of motorcycle accidents treated in the municipality.

As there is a great demand for victims and taking into account the issue of regionalization, we see patients coming into the city from neighbouring cities and states, being transferred so that they can have complete assistance, due to the Regional Hospital's structure and multi-professional team. However, even though it is the most suitable hospital to receive these victims, there is a notoriously high volume of accident victims, resulting in a greater demand for hospitalizations, costs of medication, surgical interventions and others.

According to a survey carried out in Maringà, considering the type of impact, the highest percentage was observed in the transverse collision category - 686 (35.2%). This was followed by motorcycle crashes 351 (18.0%), followed by side collisions, which were also a frequent type of impact 310 (16.0%) (OLIVEIRA, 2011).

An investigation into fatal traffic accidents carried out in São Paulo corroborates data already found in previous studies. Motorcycles were involved in 74 fatal accidents analyzed, including 7 pedestrian fatalities and 67 other types of accidents (47 collisions, 12 crashes and 8 tip-overs). Among the collisions, the most common type was the side collision, with 19 cases, followed by the rear collision (13), the transverse collision (12) and, lastly, the frontal collision, with only 3 cases (PAULA, 2008).

Pordeus (2010) analyzed the types of accidents that occurred in the capital Fortaleza, and collision stood out in 119 (56.9%) cases, followed by motorcycle crashes with 88 (42.1%) and, to a lesser extent, being run over with 2 (1%). In a study carried out by Ferreira (2009), the most common type of collision in accidents involving motorcycles was a collision (considering collision with a stationary vehicle, motorcycle with motorcycle), followed by being run over and falling.

A recent study by Tavares (2014) corroborates the data found in this study. Falls and collisions represented the main mechanism of trauma, with 455 and more than 300 cases, respectively, followed by being run over, with 37 occurrences. This data can be corroborated by this study of the local reality in Parnaiba, where the majority of accidents were caused by motorcycle collisions and falls (33.9%), followed by being run over.

It is well known that in order to stay safe in traffic, attention and care are essential. Being distracted for seconds can lead to irreparable damage, and it is of the utmost importance to be alert so that you can respond quickly to any unusual situation. Excessive speed as a contributing factor to greater damage is almost always present in accidents. Other aggravating factors can also complement a lack of attention, such as emotional or even biological factors, such as a headache or dizziness. That's why it's necessary to be prudent and recognize when it's not possible to take responsibility for driving or riding.

Paula (2008) classifies the causes of an accident in his research into three categories: those of a human nature, resulting from the actions of a driver or pedestrian; causes related to the road/environment (geometry, signage, condition, etc.) on the roads or adverse weather conditions; and causes of vehicular origin, which are those caused by faults in vehicle performance.

Also according to the aforementioned author, human factors influenced the occurrence of almost all accidents (around 99% of cases), either alone or in some cases accompanied by other factors. There were 266 indications of contributing factors for the total of 220 accidents analyzed. Speeding was the most frequent cause pointed out by the technicians (62 cases) and the use of alcohol (25 cases) also influenced various types of accidents. The recording of the incidence of alcohol is the result of heavy evidence (smell, presence of containers in the vehicle, etc.) perceived by the traffic officer (PAULA, 2008).

According to Mascarenhas (2010), when it came to the probable factors that contributed to the accidents, his study showed that 14 (46.66%) motorcyclists said they believed there was some factor that could have caused the accident. Of these, 9 (64.30%) reported poor road conditions, 3 (21.42%) pointed to poor lighting in the area, 1 (7.14%) mentioned a malfunction in the motorcycle's transmission chain, and another individual (7.14%) cited the invasion of a car in the opposite lane with a defective headlight.

Contrary to Mascarenhas (2010), Pordeus (2010) states that among the reasons given by motorcyclists for their risky behavior, speeding prevailed in 47 (52.2%) of the answers, followed by lack of attention in 33 (36.7%). When attributing responsibility for the accident to the behavior of the other person involved in the accident, the respondents recorded speeding as the main reason in 26 (54.2%) and lack of attention in 15 (31.2%) of the cases.

Similar situations were found in this study regarding the main cause of accidents. Motorcyclists attributed alcohol (26.6%) as the main culprit, followed by recklessness or lack of care (22%) and the fault of others (18%). Unfortunately, even though people know about the risks of combining alcohol and the road, they still insist on this behavior. Cities still have shortcomings when it comes to enforcement and punishment, and this opens the door to the continuation of offenses, be it the use of alcohol, driving without a license, irregular vehicles, speeding, among others. A city that doesn't enforce its laws becomes hostage to its citizens' own inconsistencies.

With regard to the condition of the victim as the occupant of the motorcycle, several studies are similar to the results obtained, as 74 motorcyclists were recorded in this study as drivers and only 35 as passengers. Tavares (2014) found that 808 individuals were in the driver's position at the time of the accident and 54 were in the passenger's position.

The same reality was found in the research by Pordeus (2010), among whom 165 (79%) were drivers and 44 (21%) passengers. This was also characterized by Palu (2013), with a sample of 168 (90.3%) drivers and 18 (9.7%) passengers. Seering (2012) discusses in his study the predominance of males as drivers (79.8%) and women as hitchhikers (73.0%), in relation to the 754 motorcycle users.

Regarding the possession of a National Driver's License (CNH), in the survey carried out in Fortaleza, there was a higher frequency of licensed drivers, with 44.2% of drivers and only 22.9% who did not have one (ALMEIDA, 2013).

This data contrasts with the local reality in the city of Parnaiba-PI and neighboring municipalities, since of the 74 drivers interviewed, only 20 (27%) were licensed, which shows a large proportion of the population without the necessary education to be driving a motorcycle or even transiting on public roads. The number of people without a license compared to the number of drivers with a CNH is alarming, and it is clear that these people expose themselves to risks and put the lives of others in danger. The lack of theoretical knowledge and the laws that underpin good conduct in traffic serve not only as a bureaucratic title, but also teach defensive driving, which can instruct in many everyday situations of risk caused by other drivers.

According to information provided by the Federal District Traffic Department - DETRAN-DF (2014), in April 2014, of the total number of licensed drivers registered in the Federal District (1,513,611 drivers), approximately 69% (1,038,133 drivers) were aged between 18 and 49. This age group corresponds to the majority of the economically active population. It is important to note that drivers must be at least 18 years old to start the licensing process (SILVA, 2014).

A survey of university students showed that more of them had a car license, with 57.28% (118) male students and 52.40% (218) female students. It is worth noting that, in both sexes, a significant number of reports of driving without a license were found, 13.11% (27) in males and 13.94% (58) in females (LABIAK, 2008).

According to Labiak, these results are worrying, as they suggest a lack of care on the part of parents, who hand over their cars to unqualified children, unaware of the seriousness of this procedure in the light of current statistics, as well as demonstrating the immaturity of young people who drive without a license while hiding from their parents.

It is important to note that according to the CBT, drivers of motor vehicles need a permit in order to travel on public roads, which is granted by means of the CNH (BRASIL, 2008).

In his study, Almeida (2013) emphasized that drivers with less than five years of driver's license had a higher gross risk of fatal accidents compared to drivers with more than five years of driver's license. This information calls into question the quality of the driver's license process in Brazil. The inexperience of new licensees shows that the rigidity of the traffic code, which provides for a provisional license of up to one year, is not enough to make them able to drive vehicles. This situation was confirmed in this study, where 45% of those interviewed with a driver's license had held it for up to 5 years.

The reality is that motorcycle drivers are unprepared and lack the skills they need to get good practice. The process carried out in a driving school alone is still not enough to make drivers fit to ride in traffic. Little experience can lead to a lack of defensive behavior.

In a survey carried out in the capital Brasilia, which looked at the behavior of motofretistas, when asked about the status of their category A license, the majority of valid answers were reported as having held their CNH for between 1 and 3 years. Of the 144 interviews, only 18 said they had been licensed for more than 10 years, which is a considerable amount of experience with this type of vehicle (MATOS, 2008).

In the study carried out by Ferreira (2009), he reaffirms the presence of drivers with less than five years' driving license. A sample of 44% had up to five years; the second sample of 39% had between six and ten years of driving licenses and those with more than ten years were only 17%.

Abreu (2010) characterized in his study the occurrence of 348 (100%) fatal victims of traffic accidents. It was observed that 94 (27%) of the victims were tested for alcohol. Of those who were tested, 11 (11.7%) victims had a negative BAC, i.e. no alcohol was detected in their blood (BAC ≤ 0.0). Of the 83 (23.8%) victims who had blood alcohol levels, 33 (39.8%) had levels lower than 0.6g/l, indicating a significant percentage of fatalities with levels below the legal tolerance limit established by the Brazilian Traffic Code.

The severity and incidence of accidents are higher at night and on weekends, which is linked to free traffic, without congestion and the use of alcoholic beverages, since the devastating effect of the combination of alcohol and high speed is well known (ALMEIDA, 2013).

In this study, a large proportion of those interviewed (31) reported drinking alcohol, especially at weekends, often on their way back from a party. Some drivers showed signs of drunkenness, although not all of them assumed that alcohol was the cause of the accident. This shows yet another irresponsible and inconsequential attitude, because as well as taking over the driving of a motorcycle, they also took on the risk of causing accidents that could eventually lead to material and physical damage, and they insisted on shifting the blame onto third parties.

A study carried out in São Paulo showed that among motorcyclists, 3% had used alcohol and in 67% of cases it was not possible to identify whether this had occurred. In the period evaluated, 63 cases of illicit drug use by motorcyclists involved in accidents were reported (RODRIGUES, 2014).

This study also confirmed the use of illicit drugs (2%), a situation revealed by motorcyclists in accidents, a common occurrence which serves as a warning, since we also have the use of other elements which cause biological alterations and deserve attention and combating by the competent authorities.

Law No. 11.705, of June 19, 2008, popularly known as the "Dry Law", was created to combat the high rates of traffic accidents caused by alcohol consumption and to punish offending drivers. But what comes into question is the role of the police in combating and intensifying these inspections. It can be seen that, despite knowing the possible punishments and consequences that the use of alcohol can bring, the population insists on combining these two weapons, putting their lives and the lives of others at risk.

With regard to the use of helmets, it is noticeable that there is still a resistance among the population to wearing this compulsory equipment, in accordance with the CTB. But it should also be pointed out that the use of this item requires care, because even if the helmet is used, it needs to be in good condition and adjusted to the characteristics of each individual, otherwise, in the event of an accident, it could cause other injuries, as was observed during the interviews in this study.

Although 55% of those interviewed said they wore helmets, during the course of the study there were motorcyclists with various injuries to the head and face, a situation suggestive of inadequate use of safety equipment.

According to Oliveira and Sousa (2003), authors in Japan concluded, through a study of autopsy records of motorcyclists, that the effective use of helmets significantly reduced the severity of head and neck injuries, but had no effect on the total severity of injuries to other parts of the body.

The research carried out by Oliveira (2013) shows that 84.58% of motorcyclists were wearing helmets at the time of the accident and 0.55% were not wearing this protective equipment, although in 14.87% of cases there was no record of this information. On the other hand, Tavares (2014) recorded in his study the presence of 43 motorcyclists who were not wearing helmets, 38 who were wearing helmets and more than 800 files analyzed did not include this information, which makes it difficult to carry out further research or even to identify the risk situation to which motorcyclists expose themselves.

Palu (2013) shows that helmets are still the equipment most used by motorcyclists, with 179 cases. However, his study also recorded the use of jackets, gloves and boots, items that can help reduce the number of injuries. The effectiveness of helmets in reducing head trauma is undeniable. Most authors not only suggest their use, but also affirm the importance of multiple, synergistic and contextualized strategies for injury prevention (RODRIGUES, 2014).

With regard to previous traffic accidents (as a driver, companion or hit-and-run driver), in the survey conducted by Labiak (2008), 66.35% (138) of male students and 53.73% (223) of female students reported previous involvement.

A second study, also carried out with young university students, corroborates these statistics. The percentage of students who had already been involved in traffic accidents was 32.8%. In the situation of being a victim of a traffic accident, the percentage of entrants was 20%, and in relation to the courses, we found relatively high percentages among physiotherapy and occupational therapy students: 57.8% and 27.7%, respectively. In relation to graduates, 12.8% had already been involved in accidents and the highest percentage was found among medical students: 55.1% (IWAMOTO, 2009).

In this study, the number of repeat victims of motorcycle accidents is notorious and significant, with 80% (40) of the victims and only 20% (10) for accidents with other types of vehicles. Corroborating this sample, around 80% of those interviewed in Ferreira's study (2009) had already suffered more than one motorcycle accident.

When people talk about greater risk when riding a motorcycle due to exposure, it's precisely because of the body's vulnerability. During an accident, with high speeds and impact with the ground or another object, trauma becomes more serious. Upper and lower limbs will be more exposed, and in many cases it is common to react by using your arms for support. Another situation that also increases the number of injuries is the lack of suitable equipment to reduce the impact and provide protection for other parts of the body, in addition to the head.

Duarte (2013) observed a predominance of injuries to the lower limbs/pelvis in 158 cases (39%), followed by 112 injuries (28%) to the head/neck and 88 (22%) to the upper limbs. These figures draw attention to the potential for complications and even lethality, since trauma to bone structures can cause serious bleeding, as is the case with fractures to the limbs and pelvis. Another warning that the study points to are head and neck traumas, which can lead to cranial and spinal trauma, requiring rare specialty care by the Unified Health System.

In this study, the lower limbs were most affected with 44 cases, followed by polytrauma with 37 records, followed by the upper limbs (16). In the capital Teresina, the same situation was found with regard to the body regions most affected in motorcycle accidents. There was a higher frequency of injuries to the

Lower Limbs (LL) with 1,055 (36%) victims, followed by Upper Limbs (UL) with 651 (23%), face with 533 (18%), Traumatic Brain Injury (TBI) 367 (13%) Neta (2012).

In Palu's (2013) findings, injuries to the extremities (upper and lower limbs) are clear and predominant, accounting for more than two thirds of the injuries (69.1%) that occurred, compared to the remaining 30.9% located in the trunk (18.6%) or the head and neck, which was the segment with the fewest traumatic injuries (12.3%).

Mascarenhas (2010) characterized the most frequent musculoskeletal injuries in his study as lower limb fractures (33.33%), followed by polytrauma (16.66%) and lower limb sprains (10%). Among facial and cranial MSDs, there was a single case of TBI (3.33%), as well as a Le Fort II fracture (3.33%).

Regarding the injuries caused by motorcycle accidents in the capital Recife, 94.7% of patients had orthopedic trauma, 5.3% abdominal trauma, and no neurological trauma was observed SOARES (2013).

In line with the findings of this study, the most common injuries were fractures (58%); followed by abrasions (30%), which can debilitate the victim for several days, leading to time off work and dependency; as well as dislocations (6.4%) and TBI (4.5%), according to the medical records of victims in the city of Parnaiba.

In a comparative study analyzing the injuries found in motorcyclists who were victims of traffic accidents and victims of other blunt trauma mechanisms, we observed that the majority of injuries diagnosed in motorcyclists occurred in the extremities (80.4%), followed by injuries in the head segment (15.5%) and, less frequently, in the thoracic (5.5%) and abdominal (3.8%) segments. When comparing injuries between the groups, we found that motorcyclists had a significantly lower frequency of extradural hematomas (0.6% vs. 2.1%), acute subdural hematomas (0.9% vs. 2.1%), subarachnoid hemorrhage (0.9% vs. 2.2%), brain contusions (1.2% vs. 3.6%), facial fractures (3.8% vs. 5.4%), and severe skull injuries (4.8% vs. 9.4%), as well as a higher frequency of diffuse axonal injury (1.6% vs. 0.7%), extremity injuries (80.4% vs. 52.2%), upper limb fractures (7.9% vs. 4.4%), lower limb fractures (7.7% vs. 5.2%) and severe extremity injuries (20.6% vs. 12.6%), (PARREIRA et al, 2010).

With regard to possible sequelae, the study shows that more than 90% of the victims had temporary sequelae, there was a small sample of three patients who suffered amputation (3%) and due to the severity of the accident, only two victims remained with permanent sequelae (1.8%). These temporary sequelae can range from simple abrasions to fractures, requiring surgical intervention, a long period of hospitalization, time off work and other problems. As for patients who have suffered amputations and permanent sequelae, a period of adaptation to the new health condition will be necessary. The absence of a limb can influence the performance of daily activities, as well as interfering with the individual's emotional state.

According to Françoso and Coates (2008), in their study of adolescent victims of traffic accidents. Of the 72 motorcyclists, 20 (27.8%) were wearing helmets at the time of the accident, while 52 (72.2%) were not. Of the 20 wearing helmets, seven (35%) had sequelae and of the 52 without helmets, 16 (30.8%) had sequelae. It was therefore observed that the group of helmet-wearers had significantly lower trauma severity score (ISS) values than those without helmets. Among those who did not wear helmets and remained with sequelae, 25% suffered severe trauma.

Senefonte (2012) highlights the etiology of extremity traumas that have led to primary amputations, where we see an almost overwhelming share of automobile accidents, followed by burns, electric shocks and iatrogenic trauma.

7 FINAL CONSIDERATIONS

After the development of this work, it was found that the situation in the city of Parnaiba, with regard to motorcyclists who are victims of traffic accidents, is in line with the national reality.

As for the research objectives, we believe that they were achieved, since we were able to describe the epidemiological characteristics of the victims, as well as covering the main causes, injuries and sequelae, as well as describing the situation of these motorcyclists, thus drawing a picture of the local situation.

It was found that the majority of motorcycle accident victims treated at the hospital were men, young people aged between 21 and 30, single, with incomplete primary education and a family income of between one and two minimum wages. Most of the accidents occurred in the state of Piaui and were victims of motorcycle collisions or falls.

The majority of motorcyclists involved in accidents were drivers and did not have a National Driver's License, while those who did have one had held it for less than five years. The regular use of helmets was identified and they considered the main cause of the accident to be the use of alcoholic beverages, although most of those involved said they were not under the influence of alcohol at the time of the accident. The victims in question had no history of previous accidents, but those who had experienced similar trauma were repeat motorcycle accident victims.

Identifying this data shows the local reality, which can have serious consequences. These range from temporary absence from work to disability or death, as well as dependency caused by irreversible sequelae. These traumas can cause social and psychological instability for the whole family.

As we have analyzed and observed during the research, we can see that motorcycle accidents have several aspects. We have a young population, with low purchasing power and schooling, who work and need an economical and fast means of transportation. Unfortunately, this population does not receive adequate instruction, because paying for a course to obtain a National Driver's License is expensive and often not in line with their reality, as they choose to buy a vehicle first and then get their license.

At the same time as these people use motorcycles for work, they also use them for leisure. And after consuming alcoholic beverages, they insist on driving this vehicle, even though they are aware of the possible penalties and accidents they could suffer or cause. What protects them and doesn't stop them from using it is precisely the feeling of impunity, because they know the local reality and are aware of the lack of inspections, so they continue to commit this infraction.

On the other hand, we identified in the study the population that has been victimized by those who have abused alcoholic substances. This is a striking and characteristic reality, both locally and worldwide. The creation of laws is of no use if they are not complied with and enforced as rigorously as they should be. As long as there is room for violations and impunity, the population will make the same mistakes again and again.

Among the measures found and cited to reduce this alarming number of victims of motorcycle accidents, we have an articulation of education, health, justice and traffic sectors. Some more urgent measures need to be adopted, such as compliance with laws, punishments and enforcement, and for these adjustments the participation of managers is necessary, who can provide the necessary support to combat offenses, as well as enforce compliance with the measures adopted.

Taking education into account, we understand that it is a long-term solution, which should be more effective precisely with children and young people. They should be taught from the outset how to behave correctly when participating in traffic, showing how bad behavior can lead to serious consequences. In addition, each individual needs to be made aware of their dangerous and inconsequential actions. Sometimes routines seen as banal can be the difference between a fatality occurring or not.

8 REFERENCES

ABREU, AM M; LIMA, JM B; MATOS, LN Use of alcohol in victims of traffic accidents: estudo do nivel de alcoholemia . **rev. Latin Am. We nurse.** São Paulo. V. 18, p. 513-20, May-Jun. 2010. Available at: < http://www.scielo.br/scielo.php?script=sci_arttext&pid=S0104-11692010000700005&lng=en&nrm=iso >. Access em: 22 Apr. 2015.

ALMEIDA, RL F; FILHO, JG B; BRAGA, J.U. *et al* . Via, homem e veiculo: risk factors associated with the gravity of traffic accidents. **Rev Saùde Pùblica** . Fortress. v. 47, n. 4, p. 718-31, 2013. Available at:

< http://www.scielo.br/scielo.php?script=sci_arttext&pid=S0034-89102013000400718&lng=en&nrm=iso >. Accessed: 14 Dec 2014.

ALVES JR, DR Como são producedas as lesões no trânso? **Associaçâo Brasileira de Medicina de Tràfego - ABRAMET** . 2014. Available at: < http://www.abramet.com.br/conteudos/artigos/lesoes_no_transito/ >. Acesso em: 30 Sep. 2014.

ANDRADE, SM of; MJ; MH P of. Terrestrial transport accidents in the municipality of the Southern Region of Brazil. **Revista Saùde Pùblica** , São Paulo, v. 35, n. 3, Jun. 2001. Available at: < http://www.scielo.br/scielo.php?script=sci_arttext&pid=S0034-89102001000300017&lng=en&nrm=iso >. Access em: 18 Sep. 2014.

ASDECOM/DETRAN-PA. Parà quer reduzier em 20% os accidentiens de trântico até 2019.

Detran-PA . Pear. Available at: < http://www.detran.pa.gov.br/news/v2/home_exibir_noticia.php?id_noticia=1682 >. Acesso em: 12 Sep. 2014.

BARROS, W. C. TS **Avaliaçâo da gravida do trauma em condutoes de motocicleta victimas de accidente de trântico no Rio Grande do Norte.** 2008. 102p. Dissertação (Mestrado) - Universidade Federal do Rio Grande do Norte. Centro de Ciências Socialis da Saùde. Graduate Program in Nursing. Natal- RN. 2008. Available em: < http://repositorio.ufrn.br:8080/jspui/bitstream/123456789/14655/1/WanessaCTSB.pdf >.

Acesso em: 14 Dec. 2014.

BRAZIL, **Brazilian Transit Code** . **Código de Tràsito Brasileiro: instituted by Lei n° 9,503, of 23-9-97** . 3 ᵃ edit it. Brasilia: DENATRAN, 2008.

BRASIL, **Código Internacional de Doenças** (V01-V99), Brasilia, 2008. Available at: < http://www.datasus.gov.br/cid10/V2008/WebHelp/v01_v99.htm >. Access em: 08 set. 2014.

BRAZIL, Ministério da Saùde. National Policy for the Reduction of Morbimortalidade por Acidentes e Violência. **Revista Saùde Pùblica** , São Paulo, v. 34, n.

4, Aug. 2000. Available in:

< http://www.scielo.br/scielo.php?script=sci_arttext&pid=S0034-89102000000400020&lng=en&nrm=iso >. Access em: 08 Sep. 2014 BRAZIL, Ministério dos Transportes - PARE Program. **Procedures for a critical local treatment of a traffic accident.** Brasilia. July 2002.

BUNS, CB Comunidade e Trànsito: Educar para o tranceto. 20th ed. Curitiba: **TECNODATA** 30P. 2006

DENATRAN **The 2014 Junho national vehicle fleet** . Brasilia. 2014. Available at: http://www.denatran.gov.br/frota2014.htm . Access em: 06 set. 2014.

DETRAN-PI Anuàrio Estatistico de Trànisto: **Registro nacional de accidentes e estatisticas de tranisto/RENAEST** . 2010. Available at: < http://www.vias-seguras.com/os_acidentes/estatisticas/estatisticas_estaduais/estatisticas_de_acidentes_no_piau i/acidentes_no_piaui_estatisticas_do_detran/anuario_estatistico_piaui_2010 >. Acesso em 09 Sep. 2014.

DUARTE, SJH; NARDES, RPMA; PENA SB; *et al.* Victims of motorcycle accidents attended by the emergency mobile service in Campo Grande, MS. **Sick Foco.** Mato Grosso do Sul. V. 4, n. 2, p. 135-139, May 2013. Available : < http://revista.portalcofen.gov.br/index.php/enfermagem/article/view/530 > Accessed: 16 Dec 2014.

FERREIRA, FF **Factores de risco em accidentes involving motorcycles in urban roads: a perception of two professional drivers.** 2009. 91p. Dissertação (master 's degree) - Post-Graduate Program in Production Engineering from the Federal University of Rio Grande do Sul. Porto Alegre. 2009. Available em: < http://www.lume.ufrgs.br/handle/10183/18974?locale=pt_BR > Acesso em: 16 Dec 2014.

FIGUEIREDO, NMA Method and Methodology in Scientific Research. 3rd **ed. Yendis** . 2008.

FRANÇOSO, L. A; COATES, V. Repercussoes sociais das sequelas fisicas em adolescentes vitimas de accidentines de tranceto. **Adolescence & Health** . São Paulo. v. 5, n. 1, p. 6-13. Março 2008. Available at: < http://www.adolescenceesaude.com/detalhe_artigo.asp?id=64# >. Acesso em: 14 Dec. 2014.

GIL, Antonio Carlos. How to develop research projects. 4th ed. São Paulo: **Atlas** , 2008.

GOLIAS, AR C.; CAETANO , R. Accidents among motorcycles: anàlise dos casos ocorridos no estado do Paranà entre julho de 2010 e junho de 2011. **Ciência saùde coletiva** , Rio de Janeiro, v.18, n.5, May 2013. Available at:

< http://www.scielo.br/scielo.php?script=sci_arttext&pid=S1413-81232013000500008&lng=en&nrm=iso >. Access em: 10 Set. 2014.

HEDA - Dirceu Arcoverde State Hospital . Parnaiba (PI). Available at: < www.heda.pi.gov.br >. Accessed: 30 Sep. 2014.

IWAMOTO, H. H; OLIVEIRA, R. C; BARBOSA, M.H.; *et al* . Traffic accidents between os studes de uma universidade pública. **Cienc Cuid Saude.** Minas Gerais. v. 8, n. 4, p. 556 562, Out/Dez 2009. Available : < http://periodicos.uem.br/ojs/index.php/CiencCuidSaude/article/view/9671 >. Accessed: 14 Dec 2014.

LABIAK, V. B; LEITE, M. L; FILHO, JSV; *et al.* Factors of Exposure, Experiência no Trânsito e Envolvimentos Anteriores em Acidentes de Trânsito entre Estudantes

Universitârios de Cursos na Area da Saùde, Ponta Grossa, PR, Brasil. **Saùde Soc** . Sâo Paulo, v.17, n.1, p.33-43, 2008. Available at:

< http://www.scielo.br/scielo.php?script=sci_arttext&pid=S0104-12902008000100004&lng=en&nrm=iso >. Accessed: 14 Dec 2014.

LIBERATTI, C. L. B. **Motorcycle accidents in Londrina: um estudo das vitimas, dos accidentines e da utilização de capacete.** 2000. 186p. Dissertaçâo (Mestrado) - Universidade Estadual de Londrina, Londrina, 2000. Available at:

< http://www.scielosp.org/scielo.php?script=sci_arttext&pid=S1020-49892003000100005&lng=en&nrm=iso >. Acesso em: 14 Dec. 2014.

LOBIONDO-WOOD, G.; HABER, J. Pesquisa em Enfermagem: Métodos, avaliação critique e utilização. 4 ª ed. Rio de Janeiro: **Guanabara Koogan** , 2001.

MASCARENHAS, C. H. M; AZEVEDO, L.M.; NOVAES, VS Lesoes musculoesqueléticas em motociclistas victims of accidents of traffic. **C&D-Revista Eletronica da Fainor** , Vitoria da Conquista- BA. v.3, n.1, p.78-94, Jan./Dec. 2010. Available em: < http://srv02.fainor.com.br/revista/index.php/memorias/article/viewFile/79/70 > Acesso em: 14 Dec. 2014.

MATOS, RH F. **Estudo exploratório das relaçôes de trabalho as a factor of influence of human behavior in traffic: the case of motofrete** . 2008. 153p. Dissertaçâo (Mestrado) - Department of Civil and Environmental Engineering , Faculty of Technology, Universidade de Brasilia. Brasilia - DF. 2008. Available em: < http://bdtd.bce.unb.br/tedesimplificado/tde_arquivos/9/TDE-2008-11-

13T153622Z- 3334/Publico/2008_RaphaelHenriqueFernandesMatos.pdf >. Acesso em: 14 Dec. 2014.

MINISTRY OF HEALTH . **Resolution N°466 OF 12 de dezembro de 2012** . Conselho Nacional de Saùde. Available to:

< http://conselho.saude.gov.br/resolucoes/2012/Reso466.pdf >. Access em: 04 Set. 2014.

NASCIMENTO, JF **Perfil das victimas de aciendas motociclicisticos atendidas em um de referencia hospital** . 2014. 48p. Trabalho de conclusâo de curso (Bacharelado em Enfermagem). State University of Piaui - UESPI. TERESINA, PIAUi, 2014.

NETA , D.S.R .; ALVES, AKS; LEÂO, GM *et al* . Perfil das ocurrences de polytrauma em condutoes motoclicisticos attended by SAMU de Teresina-PI. **Rev Bras Enferm** .

Brasilia. V. 65, n. 6, pp. 936-41. Nov-Dec. 2012. Available em: < http://www.scielo.br/pdf/reben/v65n6/a08v65n6.pdf >. Access em: 23 Apr. 2015.

NJAINE, K.; ASSIS, SG de.; CONSTANTINO, P. **Impactos da Violência na Saùde** . 2nd ed. Rio de Janeiro: Oswaldo Cruz Foundation . pp . 27-29. 2009.

OLIVEIRA, NL B; SOUSA, RMC Factors associated with the death of motorcyclists in traffic accidents . **Rev Esc Enferm USP.** São Paulo. V. 46, n. 6, p. 1379-86, 2012.

Available em: < < http://www.scielo.br/scielo.php?script=sci_arttext&pid=S0080-62342012000600014&lng=en&nrm=iso >.. Acesso em: 14 Dec. 2014.

OLIVEIRA, NL B; SOUSA, RMC Motorcycle traffic accidents and their relationship with mortality. **rev. Latin Am. We nurse.** São Paulo. V. 19, n. 2, p. 8 telas.

Mar-Apr 2011. Available at: < http://www.scielo.br/pdf/rlae/v19n2/pt_24.pdf >. Access em: 22 Apr. 2015.

OLIVEIRA, NL B; SOUSA, RMC Fatores associados ao óbito de motorcyclistas nas ocorrências de tranzato. **Rev Esc Enferm USP.** São Paulo. V. 46, n. 6, p. 1379-86, 2012. Available at: < http://www.scielo.br/scielo.php?script=sci_arttext&pid=S0080-62342012000600014&lng=en&nrm=iso >. Acesso em: 14 Dec. 2014.

PALU, LA **O custo social dos aciencianes com motocicletas e sua correlação com os indices de trauma.** 2013. 89p. Dissertaçâo (Mestrado) - Post-Graduate Program at the Surgical Clinic of the Health Sciences Sector . Federal University of Paranà. Curitiba, 2013. Available : < http://dspace.c3sl.ufpr.br:8080/dspace/handle/1884/29981 > Accessed : 14 Dec 2014.

PARREIRA, J. G; GREGORUT, F; PERLINGEIRO, J. AG *et al* . Anàlise comparativa entre as lesões encontradas em motociclistas involved em accidentes de tranceto e victimas de outros mecanizas de trauma fechado . **Rev Assoc Med Bras** . São Paulo. V. 58, n. 1, p.76-81. 2012. Available   :   < http://www.scielo.br/scielo.php?script=sci_arttext&pid=S0104-42302012000100018&lng=en&nrm=iso > Accessed: 29 Mar. 2015.

PAULA, ME B; Règio, M. **Investigaçâo de Acidentes de tranceto fatais** . Boletim Tècnico da Companhia de Engenharia de Tràfego. São Paulo. 2008. Available em: < http://www.cetsp.com.br/media/56546/btcetsp42.pdf >. Access em 19 Apr. 2015.

POLIT, DF; BECK, CT; HUNGLER, BP Fundamentos de pesquisa em enfermagem: methods, evaluation and utilization. Translated by Regina Machado Carcez. 5 ed. Porto Alegre: **Artes Médicas** , 2004.

PORDEUS, AMJ; VIEIRA, LJES; ALMEIDA, PC et al. Factors associated with the occurrence of a motorcycle accident do not perceive the hospitalized motorcyclist. **Revista Brasileira em Promoçâo da Saùde.** Fortress. v. 23, n.3, p. 206-212, Jul./Sept. 2010. Available at: < http://ojs.unifor.br/index.php/RBPS/article/view/2017 >. Access em 14 Dec. 2014.

PRADO, J. A. **Caracterização dos Acidentes de Trànsito Atendidos pelo Serviço Móvel de Urgência em Parnaiba - PI** . [Trabalho de Conclusâo de Curso]. Damn it. State University of Piaui. 2011.

ROCHA, G. da S.; SCHOR, N. Motorcycle accidents in the municipality of Rio Branco: characteristics and tendencies. **Collective health science** , Rio de Janeiro, v. 18, n.

3, Mar. 2013. Available at:

< http://www.scielo.br/scielo.php?script=sci_arttext&pid=S1413-81232013000300018&lng=en&nrm=iso >. Acesso em: 06 Sep. 2014.

RODRIGUES JM **Evoluçâo da frota de automóveis e motos no Brasil 2001 - 2012.** Rio de Janeiro. 2013. Available at:

< http://www.observatoriodasmetropoles.net/download/auto_motos2013.pdf >. Access em: 18 Sep. 2014.

RODRIGUES, C. L; ARMOND, J. E; GORIOS, C. *et al* . Accidents involving motorcyclists and cyclists in the municipality of São Paulo: characteristics and trends. **Rev Bras Orthop.** São Paulo, v. 49, n. 6, p. 602-606, Out. 2014. Available at:

< http://www.scielo.br/scielo.php?script=sci_arttext&pid=S0102-36162014000600602&lng=en&nrm=iso >. Acesso em: 29 Mar. 2015.

SANTOS, AM R. dos et al . Perfil das victimas de trauma por aciencia de moto atendidas em um serviço público de emergencia. **Caderno Saùde Pùblica** , Rio de Janeiro, v. 24, n. 8, Aug. 2008. Available to:

< http://www.scielo.br/scielo.php?script=sci_arttext&pid=S0102-311X2008000800021&lng=en&nrm=iso >. Access em: 27 Sep. 2014.

SANTOS, MG reverse; ALMEIDA , G.F. de . **Politicas Pùblicas e seus reflexos na violência dos aciencianes de tranisto no estado de Mato Grosso** . In: VI Jornada Internacional de Politicas Pùblicas. 2013. Sào Luis. Aug. 2013. Available at:

< http://www.joinpp.ufma.br/jornadas/joinpp2013/JornadaEixo2013/anais-eixo9-poderviolenciaepoliticaspublicas/politicaspublicaseseusreflexosnaviolencia.pdf >. Access em: 30 Aug. 2014.

SCHOELLER, SD et al. Caracteristicas das victimas de accidentes motociclicisticos atendidas em um centro de reabilitaçao de referencia estadual do sul do Brasil. **Physiàtrica Acta** . Santa Catarina. Abr. 2013. Available em: < http://www.actafisiatrica.org.br/detalhe_artigo.asp?id=63 >. Access em: 27 Sep. 2014.

SAUDI POLICY SECRETARIAT/MS. Programa de Reduçâo da Morbimortalidade por Acidentes de Trânsito: Mobilizando a Sociedade e Promovendo a Sùde. **Revista Saùde Pùblica** , Sâo Paulo, v. 36, n. 1, Feb. 2002. Available at: < http://www.scielo.br/scielo.php?script=sci_arttext&pid=S0034-89102002000100018&lng=en&nrm=iso >. Access em: 09 Sep. 2014.

SEERIG, LM **Motorcyclists: profile, prevalence of motorcycle use and related accidents** . 2012. 106p. Dissertaçâo (Mestrado) Programa de Pós Graduaçâo em Epidemiology. Center for Epidemiological Research. Federal University of Pelotas. Pelotas, 2012. Available at: < http://guaiaca.ufpel.edu.br/handle/123456789/1941 >. Access em 27 Sep. 2014.

SENEFONTE, F. RA; PINK, GRP S; COMPARIN, ML *et al.* Amputação primárica no trauma: perfil de um hospital da regiâo centro-oeste do Brasil. **J Vasc Bras.** Mato Grosso do Sul. V. 11, n. 4, p. 269-276. 2012. Available at:

< http://www.scielo.br/scielo.php?script=sci_arttext&pid=S1677-54492012000400004&lng=en&nrm=iso >. Access em: 16 Sep. 2014.

SILVA, AD O. C. **Alcoholic drink is a driver of motor vehicles: a dangerous combination** . 2014. 63p. Trabalho de Conclusâo de curso (Licenciatura em Quimica). Instituto de Quimica da Universidade de Brasilia. Brasilia - DF, 2014. Available em: < http://bdm.unb.br/handle/10483/8077 >. Access em 14 Dec. 2014.

SILVA, WP Profile of **traffic accidents attended by SAMU in the city of Parnaiba - PI, year 2013** . 2014. 55p. Trabalho de conclusâo de curso (Bacharelado em Enfermagem). State University of Piaui - UESPI. Parnaiba, Piaui, 2014.

SOARES, FHC **Custos diretos dos accidentes por motorcycle em um trauma hospital. September 2011 to August 2012** . 2013. 54 p. Dissertaçâo (Mestrado) Instituto de Medicina Integral Professor Fernando Figueira. Reefs. 2013. Available at: < http://pgss.imip.org.br/teses/CUSTOS_DIRETOS_DOS_ACIDENTES_POR_MOTOCICLE TA_EM_UM_HOSPITAL_DE_TRAUMA_SETEMBRO_DE_2011_A_AGOSTO_DE_2012 .pdf>. Access em 29 Mar. 2015

SOUZA AP; MORTEAN ECM; MENDONÇA FF Caracterização dos accidentes de tranceto e de suas victimas em Campo mourão, Paranà, Brasil. **Espaço para a Saùde magazine** , Londrina, v. 12, n. 1, p. 16-22, dez. 2010. Available em: < http://www.uel.br/ccs/espacoparasaude/v12n1/caracterizacao_1.html >. Acesso em: 06 Sep. 2014.

TAVARES, F. L; COELHO, M.J.; LEITE, FM C. Homens e accidentiens motociclicisticos: characterização dos accidentens a partir do atendimento préhospitalar. **Escola Anna Nery Revista de Enfermagem** . Rio de Janeiro. v. 18, n. 4, p. 656-661, out-dec. 2014. Available at: < http://www.scielo.br/pdf/ean/v18n4/1414-8145-ean-18-04-0656.pdf >. Acesso em: 29 Mar. 2015.

TDR- MOBILITY PLAN. **Integrated Urban Development Program of Catanduva:** plan diretor de mobility do municipio de Catanduva. São Paulo. 2012.

WAISELFISZ, JJ **MAPA DA VIOLÊNCIA 2013:** Traffic and Motorcycle Accidents. Rio de Janeiro. 2013.

WELTER DS; REFRIGERATOR J; BUSNELLO G. et al. Characterization of traumatic incidents attended by the fire brigade of the municipality of Itapiranga - SC. **R. pesq.: cuid. foundation Online** . Rio de Janeiro. v. 5, n. 2, p. 3020-25, Apr/Jun 2013. Available at: < http://www.seer.unirio.br/index.php/cuidadofundamental/article/viewFile/2021/pdf_732 >. Access em: 16 Jun. 2014.

9 APPENDIX

APPENDIX A - DATA COLLECTION INSTRUMENT

EPIDEMIOLOGICAL PROFILE OF MOTORCYCLISTS, TRAFFIC ACCIDENT VICTIMS, ATTENDED AT A REFERENCE HOSPITAL IN THE CITY OF PARNAIBA - PI.

Date: //

<table>
<tr><td colspan="3">Age:</td><td colspan="2">Gender: Female (   ) Male (   )</td></tr>
<tr><td colspan="5">Education
(   ) Elementary school incomplete   (   ) Complete elementary school
(   ) Secondary school incomplete   (   ) Secondary school complete
(   ) Higher education incomplete   (   ) Higher Education Complete
(   ) Illiterate</td></tr>
<tr><td colspan="5">Work:
No ( ) Yes (   ) Profession:</td></tr>
<tr><td colspan="5">Address:</td></tr>
<tr><td colspan="5">Marital status: (   ) Married ( ) Single
(   ) Divorced ( ) stable union</td></tr>
<tr><td colspan="3">Family income:</td><td colspan="2">Use of medication ( ) Y ( )N Name:</td></tr>
<tr><td colspan="3">UF of occurrence:</td><td colspan="2">City of occurrence:</td></tr>
<tr><td colspan="5">Neighborhood of occurrence:</td></tr>
<tr><td colspan="2">Type of victim:
(   ) Passenger ( )Driver</td><td colspan="2">Qualified:
( ) YES ( ) NO</td><td>Time:</td></tr>
<tr><td colspan="5">Wearing a helmet: ( ) YES ( ) NO
( ) Other ________________________________</td></tr>
<tr><td colspan="5">Indications of alcohol or other drug use
( ) Alcohol   ( ) Other drugs   ( ) Not used</td></tr>
<tr><td colspan="5">Nature
( )Run over   ( ) Collision with stationary ( ) Collision   ( )
Motorcycle crash   ( ) Not informed</td></tr>
<tr><td colspan="3">Previous accidents: ( ) YES ( ) NO</td><td colspan="2">Motorcycle: (   ) YES ( ) NO</td></tr>
<tr><td colspan="5">What was the main reason for the accident?
( ) Imprudence (lack of care)   ( ) Imperice (lack of skill)
( ) Problems on the road (signposting)   ( ) Fault of third parties (   )
Mechanical failure   ( ) Alcoholic beverage   ( )
others:</td></tr>
<tr><td colspan="5">Part of the body affected
(   ) Head/neck (   ) Face   ( )Abdomen/pelvis
(   ) Limbs SS   ( )Limbs II ( )Chest (   ) Spine</td></tr>
<tr><td colspan="5">Traumas
( ) Excoriations ( ) Dislocation ( ) Fractures (   ) TBI ()   MCT</td></tr>
<tr><td colspan="5">Prognosis/ Sequelae
( ) Temporary ( ) Permanent ( ) Amputation</td></tr>
</table>

10 ANNEXES

Annex A - Letter of Consent

LETTER OF CONSENT

I hereby declare, to whom it may concern, that we agree to carry out the study entitled **"Epidemiological profile of motorcyclists, victims of traffic accidents, treated at a reference hospital in the city of Parnaiba - Pi."**, authored by **Francisca Elineuda Morais Martins, Camila Aparecida Sousa Silva, Nayara Cristina da Rocha Oliveira.**

I declare that I have read and agree with the Brazilian Ethical Resolutions, in particular CNS Resolution 466/12, I am aware of my co-responsibility as a co-participating institution in the commitment to safeguard the safety and well-being of the participants recruited for the research, guaranteeing the necessary infrastructure.

I would like to point out that I am aware that my rights under CNS Resolution 466/12, among others, will be guaranteed:

1.   Guaranteed confidentiality, anonymity and non-use of information to the detriment of others;

2.   Use of data only for the purposes of this research;

3.   Return of the benefits obtained through this study to the people and community where it was carried out.

Place and date: *tdlYiadd - ¾Γ √5 √/ Qûtübno di*

Diretor Geral HEDA - Vitor Figueiredo Carneiro

Vitor Figueiredo Carneiro
Diretor Geral

Ht UA Hnin uba

Annex B - FREE AND DISCLOSED CONSENT FORM

RESEARCH: Epidemiological profile of motorcyclists, victims of traffic accidents,

treated at a referral

hospital in the city of Parnaiba - Pi.

INFORMED CONSENT FORM

Identification data

Project title: EPIDEMIOLOGICAL PROFILE OF MOTORCYCLISTS, TRAFFIC ACCIDENT

VICTIMS, ATTENDED AT A REFERENCE HOSPITAL IN THE CITY OF PARNAIBA - PI.

Principal investigators: FRANCISCA ELINEUDA MORAIS MARTINS, CAMILA APARECIDA SOUSA SILVA, NAYARA CRISTINA DA ROCHA OLIVEIRA.

[a]You are invited to take part in the research project entitled "EPIDEMIOLOGICAL PROFILE OF MOTORCYCLISTS, TRAFFIC ACCIDENT VICTIMS, ATTENDED AT A REFERENCE HOSPITAL IN THE CITY OF PARNAIBA - PI.", by the researchers **FRANCISCA ELINEUDA MORAIS MARTINS, CAMILA APARECIDA SOUSA SILVA, NAYARA CRISTINA DA ROCHA OLIVEIRA.**

In this study we intend to trace the profile of motorcyclists who are victims of traffic accidents and who will be admitted to the surgical clinic of a reference hospital in the city of Parnaiba, as the number of traffic accidents has been increasing every year, thus becoming a high cause of mortality and morbidity. In this context, there has been an alarming increase in accidents involving motorcyclists, which is generally due to the ease of acquisition, agility and low cost. Even with so many positive points, this type of accident causes innumerable individual and social damages, resulting in costs in hospital admissions, doctors, sequelae for the individual, disability, time off work, compensation costs and deaths.

Their participation in this research will consist of submitting to an interview and will be recorded on a form prepared by the researcher in charge, containing closed questions on socio-demographic data and the circumstances of the accident, the use or not of safety equipment and the relationship between the occurrence of the event and the suspected use of alcohol, the injured body area, injuries and sequelae will also be investigated, allowing for a more precise investigation. Data will be collected in January and February 2015, after approval by the Ethics Committee and authorization from the Dirceu Arcoverde State Hospital (HEDA).

You will not incur any costs or financial compensation. Considering the characteristics of the survey, we assure you that the risks are minimal. We will only be asking you about your sociodemographic characteristics (age, gender, race/color, etc.). It should be noted that the researchers will take care to carry out the interview at the most opportune and comfortable moment for the participant, however, as it is carried out in a hospital environment within a ward, the subject may feel embarrassed when answering the research instrument because they do not have privacy at the time of the interview.

During the interview, the subject may be accompanied by a family member or guardian to provide psychological support. If the need for assistance is perceived, the psychology and/or social services department of the institution will be asked to be present and accompanied by this professional.

The benefits will be realized through collaboration with the institution, also presented to managers, in the belief that the results can redirect strategies for preventing and/or reducing the number of motorcycle accidents, as well as improving patient care.

The privacy of the information provided and the procedures adopted will be guaranteed by the researcher in charge. The information will only be disclosed while preserving the anonymity of the patients and will be kept at the researchers' home for a period of six months.

You will be informed about the research in any way you wish. You are free to refuse to take part, withdraw your consent or stop taking part at any time. Your participation is voluntary and refusal to participate will not result in any penalty or loss of benefits.

I, ____, bearing the identity document ______________________ have been informed of the objectives of the study "EPIDEMIOLOGICAL PROFILE OF MOTORCYCLISTS, VICTIMS OF TRAFFIC ACCIDENTS, ATTENDED AT A REFERENCE HOSPITAL IN THE CITY OF PARNAÍBA - PI.", in a clear and detailed manner and have clarified my doubts. I know that I can request new information at any time and change my decision to take part if I so wish. I would also like to inform you that I agree to be photographed and that these photos may be published without my identification and with a black stripe over my eyes.

I declare that I agree to take part in this study. I have received a copy of this informed consent form and have been given the opportunity to read it and clarify my doubts.

Parnaíba, ______ from ____________ from ________

____

Name and signature of the person responsible for obtaining consent

____

Witness's name and signature

Principal Investigator: **FRANCISCA ELINEUDA MORAIS MARTINS, CAMILA APARECIDA SOUSA SILVA, NAYARA CRISTINA DA ROCHA OLIVEIRA.**

ANNEX C - DECLARATION BY THE RESEARCHERS
DECLARATION BY THE RESEARCHERS

To the Research Ethics Committee of Instituto Camillo Filho/ Sociedade Piauiense de Ensino Superior.

I, Francisca Elineuda Morais Martins, together with the other researchers, **Camila Aparecida**

Sousa Silva and Nayara Cristina da Rocha Oliveira. researcher responsible for the research entitled: **Epidemiological profile of motorcyclists, victims of traffic accidents, treated at a referral hospital in the city of Parnaiba - Pi.**

We declare that:

•	We undertake to comply with the terms of Resolution No. 466/2012, of December 12, 2012, of the National Health Council, of the Ministry of Health and other resolutions complementary to it (240/97, 292/99, 303/2000, 304/2000 and 340/2004);

•	We are committed to ensuring the privacy of the individual and the confidentiality of the information that will be obtained and used for the research;

•	The materials and information obtained during this work will only be used to achieve the objectives of this research and will not be used for other research without the consent of the volunteers;

•	The information obtained through the form at the end of the survey will be filed under the responsibility of the researchers from the nursing course at the State University of Piaui - Parnaiba campus;

•	There is no agreement restricting the public dissemination of the results, which can be made public in annals, congresses, symposia, scientific journals and other means of scientific dissemination, maintaining the criteria of research ethics, according to Resolution 466/2012-CNS/MS.

I would also like to inform you that we will only start collecting data after we have received authorization from the co-participating institution (Dirceu Arcoverde State Hospital - HEDA) and from the Research Ethics Committee of the Camillo Filho Institute/ Sociedade Piauiense de Ensino Superior.

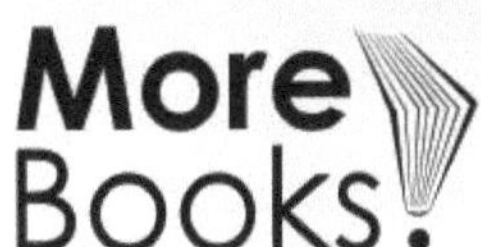

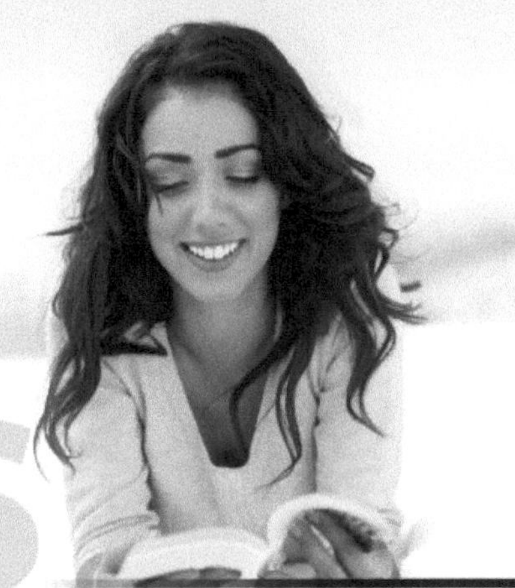

Buy your books fast and straightforward online - at one of world's fastest growing online book stores! Environmentally sound due to Print-on-Demand technologies.

Buy your books online at
www.morebooks.shop

Kaufen Sie Ihre Bücher schnell und unkompliziert online – auf einer der am schnellsten wachsenden Buchhandelsplattformen weltweit! Dank Print-On-Demand umwelt- und ressourcenschonend produziert.

Bücher schneller online kaufen
www.morebooks.shop

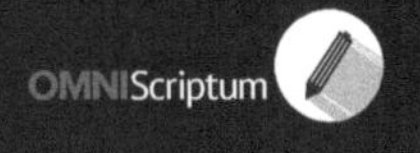

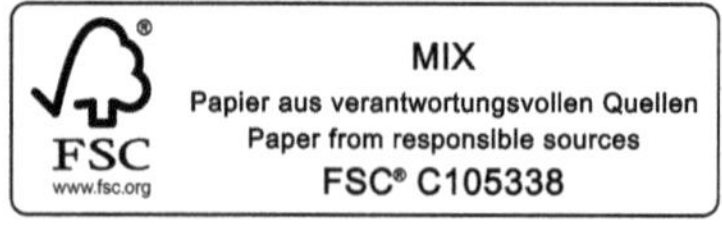

Printed by Books on Demand GmbH, Norderstedt / Germany